GET THE LOOK
2
GET BOOKED

THE MODELSCULPTFITNESS
Workbook

MODEL LOOK
MODEL SCULPT
MODEL BOOTCAMP

BY

TONI HOPPER

Note: the information in this book is for informational purposes only. It is intended for those looking to understand more about developing a healthier and fit lifestyle. As with all exercise programs you should get your doctor's approval before using this guide or any exercise routine. This workbook is best used in conjunction with a trainer or other fitness professional to begin a structured fitness regimen geared towards your needs and goals.

Disclaimer: The author assumes no responsibility for any injury that may occur as a result of attempting to do any movements, techniques, or exercises described in this workbook. Some of these exercises or activities require strenuous physical activity and a physical exam is advisable before starting this or any exercise activity. The author disclaims all liability in connection with the use of this book.

DEDICATION

After five years in the making I am happy to share with you my enormous joy for fitness. This workbook is dedicated to fellow actors, singers, dancers, performers to enjoy and contains many quick-witted innuendos and insider tips that most of us in the showbiz industry will understand.

CONTENTS

INTRODUCTION
MODEL LOOK - MODEL SCULPT - MODEL BOOTCAMP

Modelsculptfitness is a specialized fitness method for performers, actors, models, singers, and dancers based on a three phase fitness model which includes model look, model sculpt, model bootcamp. As a former talent agent with many years in the biz, my goal was to design a cool, hip, and fun fitness method for performers to use. The method is focused on improving their overall fitness level including endurance, stability, core, flexibility, and strength. It encourages them to push themselves through an endurance performance philosophy to develop a lifestyle fitness program. I also encourage everyone to get hooked 2 Modelsculptfitness and enjoy this workbook.

1 MODEL LOOK - MODEL SCULPT- MODEL BOOTCAMP
MODELSCULPTFITNESS

The Modelsculptfitness workbook is a specialized bootcamp workout and fitness workbook for actors, models, singers, dancers, performers and industry professionals. As a former Talent Agent with many years in the entertainment industry, my goal was to design a fitness method and program to address the needs of talented performers. The focus is to improve their overall fitness level including endurance, stability, core, flexibility and strength.

However, anyone who wants to look good and feel good can develop the same principles of discipline and see results. A strong commitment must be made on your part, including making smart healthy nutritional choices along with developing a workout program you can stick to M.O.D.E.L(MY OWN DAILY EXERCISE LIFESTYLE).

The average person wants to get fit, get toned and stay that way. However, if you are fortunate enough to make a living or looking to earn a living as an actor, singer, dancer, performer, you become a commodity. Industry standards are high and often demand that you look a certain way to stay at the top of your game. Anyone in the entertainment industry knows how competitive the market is, so you have to be at your best at auditions and castings. Remember, where you fall short someone else will not.

Singers need to maintain strong vocals which means strong core and good breathing

Dancers need more cardio to balance out their fitness regimen

Performers need stamina for high intensity performances

All talent can benefit from high intensity workouts that lead to better results

All talent should start with core activation and core conditioning

Proper nutrition plus a focused exercise regimen equals success for everyone. Here are a few tips to think about as you begin your journey

PERFORMERS IT'S TIME TO AUDITION YOUR NUTRITION
- Eat whole grains
- Eat green daily
- Substitute brown for white(rice, breads)
- Eat 4 -6 mini meals per day
- Think protein, protein, protein
- Increase your daily water intake
- Increase your daily fiber intake
- Eat a good breakfast daily to jump start your metabolism
- Eat less sugar and salt
- Try not to eat 2-3 hours before bedtime

M.O.D.E.L BOOTCAMP
MY OWN DAILY EXERCISE LIFESTYLE
HOW TO DESIGN YOUR BEST WORKOUT
Your workout should include the following types of exercises
1. Functional movements for everyday activities
2. Calisthenics and active rest exercises
3. Plyometric movements
4. Multi-plane movements
5. Compound exercises for large muscle groups
6. Multi-joint exercises in different directions
7. Small apparatus(bosu ball, tubes, ropes, medicine balls)
8. Free weights
9. Selectorized machines/cables
10. Body weight exercises

KEEP YOUR WORKOUT PROGRESSIVE
MAINTAIN A CUTTING EDGE WORKOUT!
Performers build endurance for your next performance
1. Alter your support base> stable to unstable
2. Alter your load> decrease and increase resistance
3. Utilize the latest in exercise equipment
4. Adjust your tempo, speed, movement, and range of motion
5. Learn how to move in all directions and planes of motion

BENEFITS OF A GOOD WORKOUT
- Better muscular endurance
- Better muscular strength
- Better muscular definition

THE MODELSCULPTFITNESS METHOD
Get hooked 2 Modelsculptfitness

PHASE 1
MODEL LOOK- Building a foundation
MODEL ABS AND CORE CONDITIONING

PHASE 2
MODEL SCULPT- Developing muscular definition
TONE AND SCULPT THE MUSCLES

PHASE 3
MODEL BOOTCAMP- Build endurance
MUSCULAR ENDURANCE MEETS MUSCULAR STRENGTH
Performers endurance performance philosophy

MODELSCULPTFITNESS METHOD BENEFITS
What you can expect
- Burn fat
- Boost metabolism
- Increase energy/increase lung capacity
- Reshape the body/sculpt and add definition
- Improve your cardiovascular endurance
- Enhance muscle tone
- Develop better flexibility
- Develop more confidence and a better body image
- Discover a new found appreciation for fitness
- Modelsculptfitness will become a part of your everyday life
- You will become more accountable for your choices regarding nutrition, health and fitness

2 THE MODELSCULPTFITNESS METHOD
3 BUILDING BLOCKS

MODEL LOOK
Start here first with model abs and core conditioning by strengthening the abs and lower back. Try to take a pilates or yoga class during this initial phase. Work on developing good posture and getting your body in proper alignment for lifting weights and resistance training in phase two.

MODEL SCULPT
Now that your body has more core strength you're ready for toning and strength training. Focus on sculpting and defining your muscles by using free weights, machines, cables, tubes, ropes, etc.

MODEL BOOTCAMP
Now it's time to move to the final phase, and your body should be ready for more challenging exercises. Your core is stronger, you've worked your muscles from many different angles. Now let's get ready to combine it all. Include high intensity bursts of cardio, active rest, calisthenics, plyometrics, isometrics, multi-joint exercises and more challenging core moves. Do these with limited rest in between sets. This helps to constantly challenge your muscles. Remember to modify all exercises as needed to suit your fitness level to prevent injury.
Always include cardio 3-5 times a week, start 20-30 minutes max
Remember to include stretching for injury prevention
Remember to consult your physician before starting this program or any physical activity
Before starting this program it's best to consult with a fitness professional. Your best investment is a personal trainer to start this program or any exercise routine or workout regimen. They can design a program geared to your goals and current fitness level.

Once you have worked with a fitness trainer, eventually you will feel comfortable to workout successfully on your own. When you have mastered a variety of exercises that are suitable for you to do, you will be ready to go through the 3 phases of this workbook. You can use the three building blocks to develop a lifetime of fun and interesting fitness sessions you can do on your own.

This workbook is for motivation and educational information only. Do not attempt any exercises mentioned in this workbook before checking with your current physician, and working with a fitness professional or personal trainer. This workbook was designed to be used with the help of a fitness trainer to help develop a program to fit your lifestyle right now.

THE MODEL SCULPT FITNESS METHOD/GOALS
  SET UP LIFE TIME FITNESS GOALS
  Here are a few tips for keeping fit for life

- Try to stay focused and motivated while you deal with life's challenges
- Keep a fitness log and The Original fitness breakdown sheet and write down your activities in the exercise log to make you more accountable
- This can also serve as a reminder of your accomplishments
- Stay inspired, don't be afraid to try new activities or sports
- Congratulate yourself for sticking to your fitness goals
- Always remember to exercise safely, don't derail your fitness plan with an injury

MSF OUTLINE-Answer these at any time during your reading
What is the Modelsculptfitness method?
Why was it developed?
Who can benefit from this program?
How can this work for you?
How to incorporate this program in your everyday lifestyle?
How to step outside your current fitness box and try something new?
How to make the best use of this workbook?

3 MODEL LOOK

MSF BASICS 101
ACTORS, MODELS, SINGERS, DANCERS, PERFORMERS
Your goal is to build core strength
Building a strong foundation starts with developing core strength, which basically means strengthening the abdominals and lower back. It is important to focus on properly aligning the body for strength training and other forms of exercise.

Any performer, especially actors, dancers, and singers who perform on stage or in front of a camera should focus on developing core strength. Core development is the foundation of exercise. This means that if the abdominals and back are strong the rest of the body can move with strength and grace. You need a strong core to perform functional activities as well as more intense strength exercises. Attention must be given to posture and carriage to get the body ready and adjusted for more dynamic physical exercises.

At this phase, exercises should include stretching along with yoga and pilates which will give the body a longer leaner look. This is the look that most models and actors seek to attain. Practicing different methods of yoga techniques is great for overall fitness and wellness. Learning to properly breathe and stretch the body is essential, it also improves health, muscle tone and strengthens the spine. At this phase try taking a class in yoga or pilates to help improve your overall wellbeing. This also gets the body ready for more challenging exercises and a better total body overall.

The Modelsculptfitness method starts with developing core strength by strengthening the abdominals and lower back. The main focus for performers is getting the body aligned for strength training along with other forms of exercise including, dance routines, tours and stage performances.

MSF METHOD/ PHASE 1 MODEL LOOK

TAKE A CLOSER LOOK AT WHAT THE WORLD SEES!

- Visual Poise-your body alignment in motion
- Model Stance-when you just stand in place
- Model Walk-how you move and walk
- How you move with grace and confidence in your daily life
- The way you sit at your desk
- The way you enter and exit a car
- The way you ascend and descend stairs everyday
- How you perform your everyday functional activities

Are you paying attention to your posture, are your shoulders back and your head held high? Remember the old adage when models walked a straight line while carrying a book on their heads. This was primarily done to help improve posture. Thankfully we are more sophisticated now and have a better understanding of body alignment.

START WITH THE BASICS

Try to correct poor posture early to encourage good form while walking on a runway, performing on stage or just doing functional exercises at your local gym. Remember, good alignment starts with a well-placed pelvis. However, most people find themselves tilting the top of the pelvis forward and swaying in the lower back. This can limit range of motion or can lead to injury during exercising or performing if not addressed.

It is important to focus on your overall alignment from head to toe, before beginning an exercise regimen. Aim to strengthen your lower abs, especially if you tend to sway in lower back. Remember, the transversus abdominis which is a deep core muscle helps to stabilize the spine. Do exercises that are great for getting the body ready. This is important for walking a runway or walking in your day to day life. Model look starts with getting the body properly aligned and ready for phase 2 Model-sculpt, which helps to sculpt the body to improve muscular definition.

HOW THE WORLD SEES YOU? HOW ARE YOU PERCEIVED?

Model look is not about your hair, your style or your clothes. It's about the way you are perceived though the eyes of others. Everyone you come into contact with will form an opinion of you based on what they see. People notice good posture and a confident body image.

Your posture and carriage give off signals to the world. Think about the way you project yourself. Do you have a strong body image? Are you giving off a confident aura by the way you walk into a room? Do you command attention at auditions or do you have poor posture, slump your shoulders and give off a dejected demeanor.

Your confidence is in your step, your swag, the way you walk down the runway, the red carpet or strut down the street. If you have never noticed this before please start now. You want to send out positive signals that you're confident and in control, whether it's going on castings or working a regular 9-5 job.

We all know that most models stand tall and erect and stand out from the rest of us. Well, we all can't be 5'10 and size 2, but we can do the best we can with what we've got. We can make ourselves appear taller and leaner by working out, standing tall, correcting our posture and tucking in our stomachs to add a more heightened look.

4 MODEL ABS AND CORE CONDITIONING
MODELSCULPTFITNESS

- Have a trainer at the gym show you their best abs moves
- Sculpt your abs, develop a defined midsection while you develop a powerful core
- Do activities to fire up your ab muscles
- Try to include abdominal development into your stretch and cardio fitness routine
- Good abs start with a strong back
- You need the proper balance of stability and strength for your back and abdominals
- Great abs come from a great total body workout plan
- Nutrition also plays a key role
- Get enough sleep and rest
- Take care of your colon
- Make sure you're getting enough water
- Make sure you're getting enough fiber
- Body fat will also determine how good your abs will look

MODEL ABS AND CORE TRAINING TRICKS
- Go clean and clean up your diet
- Try to eat natural unprocessed food
- Train and strengthen up your lower back to stabilize your core
- Focus on strengthening your core with abs and core exercises
- Work your abs consistently from all angles
- Train your rectus abdominis
- Keep track of your oblique exercises

- Do exercises with twisting movements at the waist for more definition
- Try to do cardio every day to help burn the fat
- Try a spinning or cycling class
- Challenge your abs by adding new moves every week
- Take pilates or yoga if you can

MSF PRINCIPLES - MODEL ABS AND CORE DEVELOPMENT
Principles to follow
- Correct breathing
- Proper alignment
- Focused core activation

Activate your core everywhere you go and work your pelvic floor muscles. Try to sit or stand with one hand on your lower back and the other on the lower part of your stomach, while you properly inhale and exhale. Do this a few times throughout the day.

BREAKING IT DOWN- MODEL LOOK
HERE ARE A FEW OF MY COOLEST AB MOVES TO TRY
Remember don't try these on your own, work with a trainer or fitness pro to start. In this workbook exercises are referred to as moves, and are interchangeable.

Fun moves
Abdominal hold/chair /10 sec.
Cross body mountain climber/ hold 15 secs
Side plank with leg lift
Try 3 sets of 15 reps
Try to stabilize and strengthen the back, abs and shoulders. Remember to contract your abs.

Best moves
Stacked foot plank /medicine ball
Side plank / use 2 bosu balls on each end
Swimmer /superman on stability ball
Start with 30 seconds, then 1 minute, build up to 2 minutes
1 -3 sets, keep the abs tight
Do up to 2-3 times a week

MY TOP MOVES
Hanging leg raise
Twisting oblique crunches
Abdominal bench crunches
Incline bench crunches
Start 20-25 reps/3-5 sets

GET THE LOOK 2 GET BOOKED!
TOTAL CORE SYSTEM WORKOUT
CORE STABIZATION EXERCISES
Here are a few of my basic abs & core exercises to build on
I do a couple of these each day
Select 2-3 core moves daily
You will need a stability ball to get started
Start with 10-15 reps/2-3 sets
Stability ball crunches
Reverse crunch with stability ball/floor
Vise crunch with stability ball
Stability ball rollout
Stability ball transfer/leg straddle/floor
2 leg drop with stability ball/ floor
Single leg crunch on stability ball
Side crunches on stability ball
Side plank on stability ball
Plank on stability ball
Crunch kicks on stability ball
Side leg raise stability ball /floor
Stability ball/back extension
Stability ball/ mountain climbers
Stability ball/pike
Stability ball /Russian twist/ medicine ball
Be creative and add in a few of your favorites to the list

Get the Look 2 get Booked- Total Core System workout tips
- It's important to invigorate and strengthen your core and deep abdominal stabilizing muscles
- Remember core stabilization exercises will strengthen your abs and lower back
- Understand how your internal muscles work

Transverse abdominis- these muscles help to stabilize the pelvis

Rectus abdominis- this muscle helps to flex your lower back and spine, and it also houses your potential six pack

External oblique-muscles that help you to exhale and goes across your abdomen and your lower back

Internal oblique- muscles that run deep and lets you bend your torso

TOP SHELF MOVES TO SHOW OFF - GET THAT 16 BAR CUT

Elevated side plank

Elevated plank

Elevated mountain climbers

Hanging leg raise from pull up bar

Hanging leg raise with side twist from pull up bar

Abs crunch machine

Roman chair crunches

Jackknife crunches

MODEL ABS REMIX!!!

Sculpt your abs and feel good about the way you look whether you are performing in a musical onstage or getting ready for a shoot at the beach. Learn to balance your abs/fitness workouts with your lifestyle in the entertainment industry. Put your workout on your calendar just like you do auditions, classes, and industry events.

BUILD YOUR GET THE LOOK 2 GET BOOKED CORE SYSTEM
CAST YOUR OWN CORE SESSION

Your session should focus on exercises that activate the upper, middle, lower abs and oblique muscles, also include core conditioning exercises

List your best moves
1.
2.
3.
4.
5.
6.
7.
8.
9.
10.

5 MODEL SCULPT
PHASE 2

MODEL SCULPT- BUILDING MUSCULAR STRENGTH

THE MOVES

MY PERSONAL FAVORITES

1. Walking lunges/side rotation/ medicine ball or plate
2. Push-ups /any variation
3. Pull-ups/chin-ups any variation
4. Arnold press/free weight
5. Concentration curl/free weight
6. Triceps press down/cable
7. Hanging leg raises
8. Crunches/v-sit
9. Superman
10. Side plank /underarm rotation

MY BEST MOVE HANDS DOWN
PLANK

Develop your body with one move the plank. This one move can work your core and activate about every muscle in your body at the same time. Performers, before your next audition if you have time for just one exercise do this one.

Start with 30 seconds and work up to one minute, do 2-3 times
For more of a challenge try to do different variations on alternative days
Plank it, to strengthen all the core muscles

I do a variety of planks to challenge myself. How tough do you want it?
Try the Plank Twist- one minute, 3 sets
I love this exercise!!
I know at least twenty different variations of the plank and I do them throughout the week
My go to move is the Reverse plank

BEST SCULPTING MOVES- M.O.D.E.L Z's
I like to separate my body into 3Z's
Z – refers to zones
Z 1- M.o.d.e.l UPPER BODY MSF SCULPT
Z 2- M.o.d.e.l ABS SCULPT/ CORE ACTIVATION
Z 3- M.o.d.e.l LOWER BODY MSF SCULPT

MY BEST MOVE FOR LEGS
Want fabulous legs to flaunt?
The Move- plie squat/calf raise with overhead press/ free weight
Try a couple of times a week 3 sets 12 -15 reps

Best Move abs
Want Model abs
The Move- oblique crunches-try 20 reps both sides, 3 sets
Want to activate more muscles in the abs? My best kept secret
The Move- The Hundred- yes the pilates move, do it as much as you can

Best Move back
Want that sexy back?
The Move- Plank /medicine ball- try 3 sets one minute each
My best move for lower back
Top move- Superman/stability ball-3 sets/12 reps

Best move chest
The Move- keep it simple the Push-up
Do it modified, straight up or with one hand, just do it
Do as many as you can at one time
This move works delts, triceps, pecs
For more of a challenge my pick the Decline push-up
My all-time favorite is the Spider-man push-up

More leg moves
For Hams- try lying leg curl /machine or dumbbells
For curvy calves-do calf raises anywhere and everywhere

Ranking in as one of my best moves
Walking lunge with side rotation
This one move can work many different muscle groups at one time
Hit this move with barbell, medicine ball, plate, or dumbbells

MODEL SCULPT YOUR BEST ENERGY MOVES
BACKGROUND AND EXTRAS!
I do these moves to punch up the intensity and keep my energy level up
Add these moves to your workout, or work them alone
Jumping jacks, step-ups, mountain climbers, burpees
I will do these moves anytime of the day or night when I get the urge
always in one minute intervals
My go to move is jump rope, one minute 3-5 sets
Another favorite is power skipping with jump rope outdoors

Performers you especially should add in these fun moves to your workout
Add plyometric bursts daily to your fitness program
Include fat burning moves like burpees, scissor lunges, jump squats
Top move- lateral bench hops, jump as high and long as you can

SCULPT THAT BODY!!
Add in a few of these to work the M.o.d.e.l Z's
SCULPT THE LEGS
Squats, leg press, leg curl machine, glute machine, leg extension machine
The move-deadlift barbell

SCULPT THE PECS
Bench press, pec fly machine, push-ups

SCULPT THE DELTS
Overhead press, seated rear delt raises

SCULPT THE ARMS
Chair dips, lying triceps extension, hammer curls, concentration curls

SCULPT THE LATS
Pull-ups, lat pulldown alternatives, assisted chin up machine, bent over row

6 ENDURANCE PERFORMANCE PHILOSOPHY

PERFORMERS
BUILD ENDURANCE FOR YOUR NEXT
PERFORMANCE

Performers it's important to focus on building endurance to give your overall best performance. Keep your fitness program extremely progressive. Always challenge your fitness routine or exercise regimen by adding new options to vary your workout for optimum results.

Keeping a progressive fitness program does not mean just adding more weight or reps to an already worn out routine. But adding and combining different forms of exercise, classes, sports and activities to challenge yourself to a level that you feel your best. Most of us become bored with our workout very quickly and this will make you lose focus, momentum, commitment and eventually quit.

Again, remember to focus on using the 3 phases of this workbook.
Focus on the best exercises that work muscles in each Z. Try to keep your abs engaged throughout your workout. Pick exercises for each M.o.d.e.l Z to begin your daily workout. When putting together your workout focus on the major muscle groups.

MAJOR PLAYERS- Major Muscle Groups to build your workout around
Legs
Back
Chest
Shoulder
Arms /biceps, triceps
Abs/core

For best results design your sculpting routine using different exercises(multi-joint) that can work all zones at once. Working multiple muscle groups at one time will help keep your heart rate up and burn fat. Try to sculpt, tone and tighten multiple muscle groups at once for maximum benefits.

PERFORMERS SOLUTIONS AND PERFORMERS TIPS

- Performers try to eat something 1 hour prior to rehearsal, your body needs fuel to perform at top peak performance level
- Performers keep your core tight while you are rehearsing or performing on stage
- Performers did you know that complex carbs are important to sustain muscle growth

PERFORMERS LETS PLAY DID YOU KNOW

- Did you know that 30 minutes of exercise a day three times a week can improve your overall physical fitness
- Did you know that after age 30 you can possibly lose a ½ pound of muscle each year without strength training
- After 30 some women can lose up to 20-30% of bone mass
- Did you know that resistance training is needed as a continued part of a good exercise regimen
- Did you know weight training is best when done every other day
- Did you know that plyometrics(jumping/power) can help to strengthen your joints and muscles
- Do you realize that starving the body will not get rid of body fat
- Did you know that when the muscle grows, the body will continue to burn fat
- Did you know the importance of understanding your VO2 MAX
- Did you know that running at a faster pace for a shorter distance can improve your overall stamina and endurance

QUESTION OF THE DAY

What is aerobic vs anaerobic activity?

Give three examples of each?

PERFORMERS FIT TEST KNOWLEGDE
ARE YOU SMARTER THAN...

Performers here is your research project
Look up and research the following terms
Muscle contractions
Concentric, eccentric, isometric, isokinetic
Anterior, posterior, superior, lateral, medial

Types of movement
Flexion, extension, adduction, abduction, pronation, supination

Muscle fibers
Slow twitch
Fast twitch

PERFORMERS FUEL UP FOR REHEARSAL AND PERFORMANCE
Pre/post workout fuel
Have a meal or snack before workout- 1 to 4 hours pre workout
Have a meal or snack after workout- 1 to 4 hours post workout
This will help to replenish energy, also try to eat every 3-4 hours to keep the
body in fat burning mode. Exercise builds lean muscle, which helps to burn
calories and helps boost your metabolic rate.

STEPPING OUT! STEPPING UP!
Looking to boost your metabolic rate- try this exercise move Step-ups!
Try 1-2 minutes continuous
Get the part and step it up!
Get in step and step it up!
For stronger legs- plyometric jumps, use box, platform or stepper
MY FAV- Russian step-ups

PLYOMETRICS
1. Ply jumps –box
2. Lateral hops
3. Vertical hops

BEST OF CALISTHENICS- MY PICKS
1. Cross body mountain climbers
2. High knees
3. Clapping jumping jacks
4. Squat thrust with twist
5. Running in place

When working out on your own monitor the following:
Your form
Your breathing
Your intensity(rpe)how hard you feel your body is working
It's important to understand your RMR- resting metabolic rate
This represents the amount of calories your body burns to maintain your vitals. The amount you're taking in and the amount of calories you expend.

If you are trying to lose weight or just drop a few pounds, you have to burn more calories than you are taking in. This means the number of calories you eat from carbohydrates, protein and fat.
Your body burns calories in three ways, exercise, your daily functional activities & lifestyle, and your RMR which again represents the amount of calories your body burns to maintain body functions like heart rate and breathing.

SPOTLIGHT YOUR METABOLISM
- Exercise increases metabolism
- Not eating or fasting makes the body conserve energy and slows the metabolism down
- Eating requires energy and increases your metabolism
- Hormones can effect metabolism
- Inconsistent dieting produces poor nutrition and leads to low metabolism

PERFORMERS FITNESS FOCUS- KEYS TO SUCCEED
Eat to maximize your workout
Eat frequent meals to keep your body in fat burning mode
Understanding the importance of pre and post workout fueling(eating)
Muscular fitness means muscular strength meets muscular endurance

PERFORMERS DON'T BE A STARVING ARTIST

KEEPING UP YOUR MOJO- INCREASING YOUR METABOLISM

Eat 3-5 mini/small meals throughout the day. Eating small portions keeps your metabolism at its peak and will better help you control your weight. Try eating more often, like every 3-4 hours. This keeps your body working during the day without slowing down your metabolism.

Remember skipping meals slows down your metabolism. When you skip meals your body will try to preserve itself by slowing down your metabolic rate and will store energy as fat.

Dancers and performers remember eating breakfast helps to jump start your metabolism. After a good night sleep, your body will respond to the new fuel by burning calories at a higher rate.

PERFORMERS FIT- KEEPING YOUR FITNESS LEGIT!
PRE-WORKOUT-start with one minute
Crisscross jumping jacks
Jump rope

ENCORE-BEST PERFORMERS FIT WORKOUT MOVES
Squat thrusts
Diagonal mountain climbers or vertical jumps
Jumping lunges

Calisthenics
Improves fitness and muscle tone
Push-ups, step-ups, plank jumping jacks

Best functional exercises- start here
Wall squats/ stability ball
Wall supported split lunge
Modified push-ups
Core activation
Drawing-in maneuver
Bridge
Modified plank/side plank
Bird dog

BUILDING YOUR M.O.D.E.L GYM

PERFORMERS BUILD ATHLETICISM

BEST EQUIPMENT TO INVEST IN

- Jump rope
- Resistance bands
- Bosu trainer
- Stability balls
- Free weights
- Barbell
- Foam rollers
- Kettlebells
- Medicine balls
- Suspension training equipment
- Ab roller
- Step/box
- Bench
- Heavy ropes
- Mat
- Body bars
- Sand bags
- Boxing gloves/bag
- Treadmill
- Elliptical machine
- Bike

Performers take inventory of what you currently have in your home gym. Make a list of the equipment you will need to get within the next few weeks to set up your personalized gym.

BEST EQUIPMENT TO SET UP - M.O.D.E.L GYM
   1.
   2.
   3.
   4.
   5.

MODELSCULPTFITNESS

MUSCLE MAYHEM

Performers- muscles you must know to develop a good workout

Legs- quads, glutes, hamstrings, adductors, abductors, calves

Back- latissimus dorsi, trapezius, rhomboids, serratus anterior

Chest - pectorals

Shoulder - delts-anterior, medial, posterior

Triceps- triceps brachii

Biceps-biceps brachii

Abs - internal/external oblique, rectus abdomen

Core – all muscles in the lower back and abs

Try to incorporate these muscle groups when putting together your M.o.d.e.l Bootcamp workout

THE CLUB SCENE!
HOW TO NAVIGATE YOUR WAY AROUND THE GYM
Ready to step into your next role
Performers it's time to test your machine knowledge
Do you know that weight machines can strengthen primary muscle groups
Lower body
Leg extension- quadriceps
Leg press- quadriceps, gluteus maximus
Leg curl- hamstrings

Upper body
Lat pull down- latissimus dorsi
Pec dec- pectoralis major
Overhead press- deltoids
Triceps extension- triceps
Biceps curl- biceps

PERFORMERS DON'T BE TARDY

DON'T BE TARDY FOR YOUR WORKOUT!
Get into the gym of things
Performers do you know your way around the set?
Do you know your way around the gym?
Ask a fitness director, manager or personal trainer for help, most gyms offer complimentary newcomers 1st workouts to get familiar with the facility. Here is a basic selectorized machine workout, adjust your weight accordingly.
Leg press- quads, glutes
Leg curl- hams
Calf machine- calves
Lat pulldown- back
Chest press- chest
Shoulder press- shoulders
Arm extension- triceps
Arm curl- bicep
Ab machine- abs
Try 2-3 sets of 12-15 reps 2-3 times a week to start

SHOWTIME- DEVELOP YOUR LIST OF EXERCISES
-
-
-
-
-

SELECTORIZED MACHINES- DEVELOP YOUR LIST
-
-
-
-
-

Remember to get a description of proper form and technique from a fitness professional before attempting any exercises in the workbook.

PERFORMERS/ PRE AND POST WORKOUTS
Breakdown a list for your pre-workout(warm up phase)
-
-
-
-
-

Breakdown a list for your post-workout (cool down phase)
-
-
-
-
-

PRE-AUDITION PREP
Do 10-15 minute pre-audition workout to get your energy up and show some confidence
Try jumping jacks, jump rope, pushups or running in place

POST AUDITION PREP
Try taking a class like cycling or boxing to work off tension and stress

GET PREPPED FOR THE BIG ONE
What to do the night before a big audition?
Bicycles/abs
Bicycles help to strengthen all the core muscles and is great for your body stability and abdominal toning

Performers fit focus- two components
1. Muscular strength refers to the maximum amount of force a muscle or muscle group can exert at one time. How much weight a muscle can move.

2. Muscular endurance refers to the amount of times a muscle or muscle group can repeat the same movement

PERFORMERS TIPS- STEP INTO YOUR FITNESS ROLE
1. Exercise builds lean muscle that helps to burn calories faster than fat does and will raise your metabolic rate over the long haul
2. By building and maintaining muscle you will burn more calories
3. Strength training and aerobic activity increase energy
4. You need aerobic activity to burn calories
5. You need resistance training to build more muscle

ENDURANCE FOR THE PERFORMANCE

Building blocks to help you on the road to more stamina and endurance
- Remember don't be a starving artist
- Make sure to keep your body fueled all day
- Don't skip meals
- Keep your energy level high by eating nutritionally balanced meals and snacks during the day
- Constantly remember to audition your nutrition
- Don't be a workout dropout
- Continue to build up your endurance
- Focus on your endurance/performance philosophy

PERFORMERS PEAK PERFORMANCE
Performers, dancers and entertainers have hectic schedules while touring and need stamina to perform on stage for many hours non-stop. Make sure to get enough cardio and strength training to stay at the top of your game.

Top performance tip- My choice is kickboxing
Performers kickboxing can help build greater endurance if done on a regular basis. It can also help your body become stronger by continuous repetitions of kickboxing techniques that will give you more stamina.

Performance Benefits
- Your lower body will become stronger from the constant repetitions from doing kicks
- Your upper body will become stronger and have more definition from the constant repetition from doing punches
- The combination of doing kickboxing is both anaerobic and aerobic. You burn calories as you increase your energy level

DON'T BE A WORKOUT DROPOUT

TOP TIPS FOR ACTORS, DANCERS, PERFORMERS

1. Get started the right way. Pick a time, date, and location to begin your fitness program
2. Plan out how often you realistically can stick with your fitness plan
3. Plan out a schedule for a 6 week fitness program
4. Define your fitness goals, list 3 things you wish to gain from your workout
5. List your top 5 reasons why you failed to stick with a fitness regimen in the past
6. Focus on fitness not food
7. Make fitness a part of your daily exercise lifestyle
8. Discover your inner fitness guru
9. Keep up the pace and keep feeling the burn, make sure to work up a sweat and feel your muscles working
10. Keep your workout progressive

BUILD YOUR CHARACTER/ BUILD YOUR STRENGTH

The importance of strength training for actors, dancers and performers is necessary. Strength training is crucial for dancers and performers to develop the best body they can. Actors and models want to build lean muscle to look natural, good and healthy on camera, on screen and in photos.

Remember, the camera can add 10-15 pounds depending on how close up the shots are and depending on the angles. Your workout requires strength training a few times a week to lean you out.

THINK OUTSIDE THE CARDIO BOX

Understanding the importance of cardiovascular exercise
Cardiovascular exercise helps to increase lung capacity for more energy, and improves stamina. This is important to have energy while giving a live onstage performance or just running to castings, auditions and rehearsals.
Actors and entertainers try to walk as much as possible. In NYC walk quickly to keep your heart rate up instead of taking the train. If you do this 3-4 times a week, you will be getting in some of the cardio you need.

Take the stairs up and down as much as possible, on the way to the subway, at work or in the building where you live. Taking every additional extra step counts to keep your energy level up.

PERFORMERS CHEAT SHEET!!!!

DANCERS BOOTCAMP TIPS

Remember great alignment starts with a well-placed pelvis

Try not to force your turnout too much

A dancers #1 priority is to stay injury free

Pre-planning your workouts can reduce injuries

Make sure you're getting sufficient calories each day

Make sure to eat mini meals between rehearsals and classes

Don't critique your body by comparison to other dancers

Try not to over train your body

Try to take other fitness classes

Dancers try to get in 20 minutes of cardio 3-5 times a week

SINGERS BOOTCAMP TIPS

Master your vocal cord function

Sing from your source of power, your diaphragm

Focus on breathing and try to expand your vocal range

Develop harmony and ear training

Take care of your diet and vocal health

Singers have special needs for onstage performances, you need trained vocals so focus on core exercises for proper breathing. Also, try to punch up your stamina by developing a strong cardio regimen.

ACTORS BOOTCAMP TIPS

ACTOR-FITNESS-SWAG TIPS

Since the camera can add pounds at different angles focus on good posture, strong presence and having an overall healthy look and tone. Getting and keeping a fit and natural look that shows good muscle tone is what you should strive for.

Eat a healthy breakfast to start you day

Eat healthy foods to help with memory and brain function

Learn your lines, go over your sides and jump into character with a boost of energy

Actors revamp your workout and your resume at the same time

Actors bump up your fitness and add in new skills, hobbies and physical training

Start adding to your resume by including more sports, skills and hobbies that can make you more marketable for casting projects

Make a list of new activities or sports you want to add to your resume over the next few months like, kayaking, skating, fencing and more

COOL-ACTOR-FITNESS-SWAG TIP FOR ON CAMERA

Improve your on air persona by noticing how straight and erect more experienced actors stand, angle and project themselves on camera. They do not appear nervous or uncomfortable being in front of the camera. Many seem to radiate a certain self-assured on air quality. Make sure to work out during the week to have more body confidence when it's time to face the cameras.

OPENING ACT
JUMP INTO FIT-ACTING 101
GETTING STARTED ! EXERCISE MOVERS AND SHAKERS

- Walking
- Lunges
- Squats
- Row
- Back extension
- Push-ups/ modified
- Pull-ups/ modified
- Reverse fly
- Triceps dips
- Bicep curls
- Bird dog
- Plank
- Crunches /variations

Use free weights as needed
Start with 3 sets of 12-15 reps

SCENE 1-FEMALE FITNESS PERFORMANCE!

Did you make the cut? Here are a few moves to build upon
Model sculpt firmer more well defined arms

- Triceps overhead extension/ free weight
- EZ-bar lying triceps extension/ bench

Want more definition? Build the outer head of the tricep

- Triceps press down / cable
- Crossover chest extension/ free weight

BUILD A MIGHTY BICEP
- EZ bar curl/ standing
- Bicep curl/incline bench free weight
- Preacher curl

Are your biceps still a bit flat? No definition?
You need to build your biceps peak
My best sculpting move
- Concentration curl/ free weight

Second runner- up
- Crossover cable curl

 For each exercise start with 3 sets of 12 reps

KEEP THE PECS IN CHECK!
Bench press/ barbell
Incline press /free weight
Pec fly/flat bench/ free weight
Try 3 sets of 12 reps

KEEP THE SHOULDERS STRONG!
Rear delt raise/free weight
Lateral raise/ free weight
Seated overhead press/ free weight
Try 3 sets of 12 reps

BRING THE SEXY BACK!
Seated cable row/ machine
Lat pulldown/ machine
Barbell row
Inverted row
Try 3 sets of 12reps

LEGS, LEGS, LEGS!
Squat /barbell or smith machine
Lunge/ barbell or smith machine
Try 2-3 sets 15 reps

SCENE 2-MALE FITNESS PERFORMANCE CHALLENGE!
Go hard core! Top moves to make your muscles shake!

- Ply jumps/high box
- Jump squats/barbell
- Single leg barbell lift
- Split squats/smith machine
- Pull-ups/single arm pull-ups
- Push-ups with claps
- Push-up/medicine ball/single arm push-up
- Single arm, single leg plank/medicine ball
- Bench press
- Deadlifts
- Arnold press
- Biceps curl/barbell
- Single arm triceps press down
- Weighted dip/triceps dip with plate
- Sit ups/eagle spread
- Incline leg press/Incline hack squat machine

Try some of these muscle builders to develop a 30 minute circuit. Feel free to add in some of your own top moves to balance it out, just remember to adjust the load to continue to challenge your muscles.

GETTING IN A GOOD STRETCH BEFORE AND AFTER
Work that body, now stretch that body!

It's important to stretch before or after a workout to help prevent injury. Stretching helps the body cool down after a workout and improves joint flexibility. There is no better feeling after a workout than to stretch and elongate the muscles activated during your exercise routine. While doing stretches before your workout is a great way to warm up the muscles. You can warm up with static stretches and cool down with dynamic stretches.

Performers you can also include stretching in your workout routine. Your body needs to recover after a grueling rehearsal and stretching can help. Remember to include stretches for quads, hamstrings, calves, back, chest, neck, shoulder, biceps, triceps, etc.

7 AUDITION YOUR NUTRITION

PERFORMERS HEALTH AND NUTRITION BASICS 101
See your doctor or health care specialist annually
Check for food allergies and discuss physical or health related issues
Learn the keys to solid meal planning
Learn how to mix and match from various food groups
Energy in vs. energy out, try to burn more calories than you take in
Always make healthy food choices
Don't skip meals in the am
Try to eat before a training session, rehearsal or performance
Try not to wait too long to eat after your workout
Keep yourself hydrated all day long

TALK TO MY AGENT! BUT FIRST TALK TO MY DOCTOR!
Don't forget the importance of doctors and other medical professionals to help you understand what's going on with your body at different stages of your life and career. Your physician can help you understand metabolic and hormonal balance, and discuss food options that are best for you based on your current and past medical history. Also, ask about the level of your daily physical activities from intense endurance training to muscle building workouts.

Here are a few signs your body may not be getting proper nutrition
Lack of energy and focus
You're tired all the time
Constant bloating or belly fat
Bone weakness which could lead to osteopenia or osteoporosis

MAKE AUDITION NUTRITION PART OF YOUR M.O.D.E.L
Take the quiz below- test how well you're nourishing your body
Essential groups of nutrients
Protein
Carbs
Fats
Water
Vitamins

Get your vitamin regimen in gear
Give 2 examples of foods rich in the following
Vitamin A
Vitamin B
Vitamin C
Vitamin D
Vitamin E
Vitamin K

Give 2 examples of the following
Complex carbs
Simple carbs

Give 2 examples of
Polyunsaturated fats
Monounsaturated fats

Give examples of the following food groups
Grains
Vegetables
Proteins
Fruits
Dairy
Oils

DEVELOPING HEATHY SOCIAL NETWORKING SKILLS
Tips for dining out! Develop a restaurant game plan
Limit soups, appetizers and deserts
Focus on nutritious entrees and heathy salads
Try not to order anything with gravy or sauce
Order broiled or grilled
Always request steamed vegetables

GIVE YOUR MEAL THE GREEN LIGHT! GO GREEN!
Try these leafy greens
Kale, spinach, collards, cabbage
Add a few more of your own favorites to the list

TIME TO RECAST YOUR COCKTAIL
Some cocktails have more sugar than alcohol
Remember they are loaded with hidden calories
When in doubt go for sparkling water or club soda with lemon and lime

HEALTHY CHOICES! SHOWBIZ CHOICES!
You make decisions and choices about your career every day
Why not do the same for your health and wellness
Create new tips for a healthier you
Make a list of 5 new healthy choice tips to follow
Remember the components to a healthy M.O.D.E.L regimen is good nutrition, cardio/aerobic activity and continued resistance training

PERFORMERS IT'S TIME TO GET TO KNOW YOUR BODY
WHAT ARE YOUR STATS

BODY FAT
Males and females should know their body fat percentage and understand how it relates to your overall health

BMI
Know your body mass index. Understand your height to weight ratio and its effects

WAIST CIRCUMFRENCE
Know your measurements and health risks associated with them

GET YOUR BODY FAT TESTED
Bioelectrical impedance testing
Body fat analyzer
Skin fold caliper testing

ASSESS YOUR ASSETS
Fitness assessments include the following areas
Body composition, flexibility, sit and reach test, muscle endurance, cardio endurance

M.O.D.E.L MEASUREMENTS

HOW DO YOU MEASURE UP

Take your measurements with a measuring tape every 3-4 weeks to check results and see if you are adding muscle. Models you know how important measurements are for fittings and wearing sample size clothes. Actors and performers make sure to keep up with your measurements for wardrobe and costume fittings especially for stage and theatrical performances.

Get friendly with your measuring tape
Seven body part measurements
Chest
Shoulder
Right arm
Waist
Hips
Right thigh
Right calf

MY PERSONAL HEALTH AND WELLNESS GOALS
It's time to take inventory of your entire health, nutrition and fitness
Prepare a list now and breakdown your nutritional goals
Deconstruct your nutrition to suit your dietary needs. This should be a sample of food groups and any dietary restrictions. It is important to focus on nutritional value and protein to build heathy lean muscle.

ARE YOU READY FOR THAT IMPORTANT GO-SEE?
That means go see your doctor asap to get a check up
Don't overlook this important aspect to maintain proper health and a strong body. Also see a nutritionist to make sure your nutrition is on point.

8 MODEL BOOTCAMP
PHASE III
INTRODUCING M.O.D.EL. BOOTCAMP

The concept of M.O.D.E.L bootcamp was designed to be used as a power circuit training workout to provide a one stop total body exercise session, combining strength training and cardio in a single workout. It helps to reduce bodyweight, burn fat and build lean muscle. It can also improve your overall strength and endurance while adding variety to your fitness regimen and routine. This is a great way to sculpt and tone the body.

Your goal is to design your own M.O.D.E.L bootcamp and power circuit training session by incorporating exercises to improve power, speed, endurance, stamina, flexibility, functionality, strength, balance and agility. Try to use the bootcamp model to build strength and endurance and eventually help tone and sculpt a better body.

BENEFITS OF M.O.D.E.L BOOTCAMP
Bootcamps are now a new exercise of choice for many people. It generally combines a mixture of cardio and strength training moves. Many include explosive and ballistic moves like jumping, push-ups, running drills, mountain climbers to name a few, along with many variations to accommodate the level and goal of the bootcamp.
Many people feel a sense of pride after doing this intensive work out because they are doing many of the same moves that many athletes do. In addition, they can easily duplicate the same exercise moves on their own and feel quite at ease.

M.O.D.E.L/MY OWN DAILY EXERCISE LIFESTYLE BOOTCAMP

It's time to step up and design your own circuit training plan/bootcamp
Step into your first starring role- featuring you

You pick the time – Start with a 30 minute bootcamp circuit, three times a week. As you progress and your fitness level improves, you can increase the amount of time, intensity and the number of days per week you can perform the circuit.

You pick the place- circuit training can be performed in a gym, your home with a simple home set up, backyard, park, your office or any outdoor location.

Remember, as you design your bootcamp keep up a brisk pace moving rapidly from one exercise to the next. The entire session works your cardiovascular system. Your M.o.del bootcamp session should start with a light cardio warm up of your choice, stretching and a cool down phase. Start your bootcamp with your top 5 to 8 strength exercises targeting major muscle groups and complete them one after the other with only a short rest in between. Your bootcamp can consist of a total body workout or just the upper body, lower body, or core exercises. Also, you can vary the program to add variety to your workout.

M.O.D.E.L BOOTCAMP
PRE-PLANNER FOR MID LEVEL NEWBIE/INGENUE

Create a 10-30 minute circuit
Pre-plan and write down your bootcamp exercises
Pick 5-8 exercises to do
Remember to include major muscle groups, abs and core and active rest exercises
Change up your bootcamp by adding new exercises
Use balls, bands, kettlebells, free weights, heavy ropes, bars and more
It's important to keep up a brisk pace moving from one exercise to the next with little rest in between

SWITCH IT UP! EXPAND YOUR RANGE!

You need to switch up your workout every 3-4 weeks
- Develop a brand new circuit of exercises
- If you can do it add in more plyometrics like box jumps
- Try the latest in suspension training
- Alternate your rest day
- Don't make your bootcamp to easy
- Keep your workout challenging

- Do your bootcamp 2-3 times a week, at home, work, park, beach
- Do other types of fitness and activities on your off days like cycling, sports, classes, swimming, running, hiking, skiing
- Give your body one full rest day during the week

GET INTO THE GROOVE-GO MULTI- JOINT

This means working three or more muscle groups at one time. These exercises are very challenging and should not be done as a beginner of a strength training regimen. Also, try to modify exercises to your ability and preferably under the guidance of a personal trainer to start. Again, these exercises can be very strenuous and should not be done on your own but with the help and of a fitness pro.

Always begin a good fitness program with the help of a trainer or fitness coach. They will help you determine load, reps, sets and sequences. They will also check your form, breathing, and intensity during your workout. Again, once you have acquired better knowledge of basic exercises, you can proceed on your own to build your M.o.d.el Bootcamp program.

DESIGNING YOUR M.O.D.E.L BOOTCAMP MOVES

Here are a few moves from my personal fitness playbook
Add in a few of these along with your own favorites

MARQUEE FITNESS LINE UP-TOP WARM UP MOVES
GET THE HEART PUMPING

High knees
Jumping jacks
Lateral box jumps
Alternating lunges
Jump squats
Explosive high steps
Inchworm
Mountain climbers
Walking push-ups
Plank push-ups
T-push-ups
Barbell lateral jumps
Burpees

TOP BILLIING-TOP PLY-MOVES TO JUMP UP YOUR FITNESS
Step-ups/side step-ups
Scissors Jump lunges
Ply jumps/box
Lateral side step-ups/bosu ball
Stability ball push-ups
Jump rope/single foot hops
Hurdle jumps
Bosu ball burpees

GO ISO
No bootcamp can be complete without mixing in isometric moves. My live fitness events are built around isometric exercises. I have always included isometric training at my two top fitness and net-working-out events Model Bootcamp Rocks and The Model Talent Fitness Party Workout.
Isometric exercises are not easy and can be quite challenging. These exercises are performed without changing the length of the muscle. Many yoga and pilates moves are isometric in nature.

TOP ISOMETRIC MOVES TO ADD TO YOUR WORKOUT
Forearm plank/ side plank
Prone cobra
Isometric push-up
Isometric low plank
Wall sit variations
Static lunge
Squat hold
Wall push-up
Pull-ups
Shoulder raises
Dead hang

BENEFITS OF ISOMETRIC TRAINING
1. Isometric moves help to condition and strengthen the muscles
2. Isometric moves will give you more control over your body
3. It helps to improve your posture and body alignment
4. Many of the exercises are used for injury rehabilitation
5. It helps to develop lean muscle
6. Can help to improve bone density
7. Will help with endurance ability
8. Will activate major muscles in the body
9. Iso exercises don't require equipment
10. No specific location needed and can be done anywhere

Isometric exercises can also be used in your workout in between other exercises. Talk with your trainer to see how to best incorporate these moves into your M.o.d.e.l Bootcamp program.

GET BOOKED! BOOK YOUR WORKOUT TIME EACH WEEK!
CREATING YOUR LIFETIME CUTTING EDGE FIT PROGRAM
Start by developing a M.O.D.E.L weekly program
Cardio 3-4 times a week / 20-30 minutes max
Abs and core conditioning- daily
Strength training 3-4 days a week
Bootcamp workouts- 2-3 times a week

Keep your own work out progressive and mix up your exercises, sports, and activities routine. Remember to keep your workout interesting so that you yourself will want to show up. Book and schedule yourself in everyday for your workout include day, time, location and specifically what you will be doing ex. cardio, strength, and a list of exercises like jacks, planks, abs, jogging, etc.

Try to look forward to enjoying your workout, most people are bored that's why they don't show up or forget to go to the gym or ditch their plans to work out on their own. You must make an appointment with yourself to exercise and keep your motivation going.

PLEASE DON'T BE A WORKOUT DROP OUT!!

REASONS WHY PEOPLE FALL OFF THEIR EXERCISE REGIMEN
1. They are not motivated
2. They are bored with their exercise routine
3. They have not seen any results
4. They don't know what to do during their workout
This sets up the cycle to fail or quit exercising all together, hence becoming a workout drop out

MAKING YOUR WORKOUT STICK!
My suggestion is to focus on getting your body strong and healthy. Develop a strong commitment to get fit by sticking to your workout so you have a better understanding of why you need to make fitness a part of your lifestyle. Then you can begin to conquer your daily health and nutritional needs. Don't wait to start an exercise program. Use fitness to jump start your goals to overall fitness, health and wellness.

TURN-UP!!!

MODEL BOOTCAMP ROCKS!!!

THE FITNESS BREAKTHROUGH FOR BUILDING ENDURANCE

Performers build up your endurance for your grandest performances and showcase your athleticism. This is the culmination of everything you've worked so hard for. It's time to up the intensity of your next workout and breakthrough all fitness barriers and achieve your long term fitness goals.

Now that you've mastered the basics of bootcamp it's time to kick it up a notch. Start by rocking your most challenging strength, core and body weight moves and combine them into a personal power bootcamp session

TURN-UP!!!!
ITS TIME TO TURN UP THE INTENSITY
Rock your core to its foundation with your toughest abs moves
Push yourself to the max
Pick your own combination of upper and lower body moves and include multi-joint exercises

MODEL BOOTCAMP ROCKS- BREAKDOWN
Do 3 -5 rounds of any five exercises for 1 minute up to 2 minutes each moving quickly from one exercise to the next with no rest. After each round include 1-2 minute core phase, by doing 1-2 minute plank in any variation. Restart the next round.

This formation is used in my live fitness event "MODEL BOOTCAMP ROCKS" and is quite the challenge for performers. It's a continuous fitness flow that works and fires up the muscles while keeping the endurance level at a good pace.

Sample : jumping jacks, push-ups, cobra, lunges, triceps dips
Do each exercise for 1-2 minutes with no rest, now include your core phase for 1 minute. Finish and proceed to next round with no rest.
The most important part is to include the core phase to work your core muscles and make you work harder as your body starts to fatigue.

Now build your own and rock it out! Make your workout rock!
Try 3 rounds to start without rest using the core phase as a resting and reset phase. Add more rounds and exercises as you progress to make it more of a challenge.

STUNT TRAINING ANYONE ?

AGILITY, STUNT AND SPORTS TRAINING FOR PERFORMERS

Actors and performers be prepped for your next live stunt!
As an actor you never know what your next live stunt on camera will be or what is required for your next role. So when in doubt always be prepared. Keep in tip top shape by being active and participating in sports and other physical activities. Up your training for both indoor and outdoor activities, sports and fun.

Try these to strengthen up your core and upper body

- Ziplining
- Kayaking
- Rock climbing

Looking to build a stronger lower body
If I had to pick one sport to show off a model sculpted body make it beach volley ball. This is a great workout and builds superb leg power. You can enjoy volley ball in the gym or on the beach year round.

I also use this leg builder at least once a week in my workout
Clock lunges- moving your legs to points on a clock works and strengthens your legs from every angle. This helps to get your body in tip top shape.
Also try reverse lunges, and walking lunges with high kicks

Best performance move for performer- The Bleacher Workout
Performers if you're going on tour or need to get your stamina high this will help. Try running bleachers up and down continuously non-stop for 3-5 minutes. If you need to modify try just briskly walking up and down the bleachers to get your heart rate up.
Bleachers-one move 3 variations

- Bleacher step-ups
- Bleacher ply jumps
- Bleacher lunges

Repeat as many times as you can before resting

Top performance activities you can perform any time to get into the groove
Surfing, hiking, swimming, cycling, mixed martial arts, sprinting, jogging

ACT- BI-COASTAL

ACTORS KEEP YOUR FITNESS COOL & BI-COASTAL
NY/LA

BEST ACTION SEQUENCE PLAN IN NYC
1 WALKING/ # 2 JOGGING
Try to do this as much as you can daily
- Walking/crosstown
- Climbing /stairs(subway)

Coolest place in NY to walk, jog or just profile is Central Park

HEY LA
BEST ACTION SEQUENCE PLAN LA STYLE- SWIM
Best spot in LA to workout is the beach
You can do the coolest workouts on the beach as well as a variety of water sports to keep your fitness in check
Plan to look good and stay in max shape year round no matter what side of the coast you're on

GETTING A LONGER LEANER LOOK YEAR ROUND

Tips from "THE MODEL TALENT FITNESS PARTY WORKOUT"
- Aim to build more muscle so your body will appear tighter. This will give you a more toned look.
- Aim to burn more fat by doing cardio
- Aim to increase stamina by doing bootcamps, circuits, and HIIT workouts
- Include stretching, yoga, and pilates to improve your core strength and flexibility which can also give you a longer look
- Make sure to warm up before exercising
- Make sure to use good form when exercising
- Make sure you don't over train
- Do not get into an exercise rut
- Get enough sleep at night
- Stay hydrated all day long
- Pay close attention to your nutrition

MAJOR RECAP – MAIN POINTS TO REMEMBER

MODEL LOOK- focuses on abs and core activation

MODEL SCULPT-focuses on sculpting and defining your muscles through strength training

MODEL BOOTCAMP-focuses on both muscular endurance and muscular strength. This is a high intensity circuit training workout combining strength, cardio, calisthenics, body weight, multi-joint exercises and more

USING THE M.O.D.E.L BOOTCAMP PROGRAM
Building my own daily lifestyle fitness program

Fitness Breakdowns- selecting your own weekly top picks
Cardio- 3-5 times a week, your choice
Warm up and cool down/stretching-your choice

Select at least one action activity, class or sport to do 1-2 times a week like cycling, tennis, volleyball, swimming, group fit class, spinning
Performers in addition add in time for rehearsals, dance classes, stage work

CASTING YOUR M.O.D.E.L BOOTCAMP LIFETIME PROGRAM

PHASE 1 – Model Look- Model abs and core conditioning exercises
3-5 times a week or every day
Select your top abs and core exercise moves to perform
Do alone or combine with Model Sculpt(Phase 2)

PHASE 2- Model Sculpt- toning and strength training exercises
Strength train minimum 3 times a week
Select your top total body exercises to hit every muscle group be sure to include free weights, cable apparatus, machines
Do alone or combine with Model Bootcamp(Phase 3)

PHASE 3- Model Bootcamp- high intensity exercises
1-2 times a week, in addition to strength training
Put together a high intensity total body workout to build strength, stamina, endurance and burn calories

DID YOU BOOK IT
BOOKING YOUR BOOTCAMP!!!

Create your own circuit and build your M.o.d.e.l bootcamp workout

Combine with Phase 1, Phase 2, and various multi-joints movements

Calisthenics, plyometrics, isometric exercises, sports drills, active rest and extreme cardio

Pick 6-8 exercises hitting all major muscle groups add in bursts of cardio and go hard for 30 minutes. You pick your own exercises and do with limited rest in between sets, do three rounds. Remember your warm up and cool down phase. Push yourself bootcamp style, work yourself hard and don't let up.

Follow up with other fitness activities on your off days like cycling, sports, classes, swimming, running, hiking, skiing, and most water sports

9 FITNESS FOR THE INDUSTRY PRO

As a former Talent Agent, I'm dedicating this section to all the industry people in the entertainment biz who are mostly confined to a desk six to eight hours straight. I know firsthand how difficult it can be to fit in an exercise program during such a hectic day. I started early with breakdowns, being at the desk for long periods of time, constantly on the phone with managers, casting directors and producers while steady on the computer. This doesn't leave much time to work out or stretch your muscles during the day. Tight hip flexors and hamstrings usually result from this and you may even experience back problems. Your goal is increase your mobility as much as you can. Try to take short mini breaks during the day and do stretching at your desk.

INSIDER TIPS
Don't hunch over your desk, maintain good posture by keeping your back and shoulders resting on the chair
Keep your computer at eye level so not to strain
Make the owner of your agency invest in chairs with an arm rest
Try to keep your feet flat on the floor, too much twisting can throw off your alignment
Activate your core all day by drawing in those abdominal muscles
Remember to take your daily walk
Don't skip your lunch break(I know what lunch break)
Take a 15-20 minute walk to boost your energy level and increase your heart rate

Your main goal is to concentrate on 3 key areas of development
- Strength training to build and retain muscle
- Building core strength
- Cardio, cardio and more cardio. By all means get more walking into your day

Try to walk as much as possible and move briskly as you go about your day to get in as many steps as you can. You can even have light weights or grips at your desk to use at any point during your day.

IN OFFICE MOVES AND SHAKES
Try a few of these on your down time

Director's Chair Squats
Try 3 sets of 10-15 low and slow squats using your chair. This will help to strengthen your lower body and improve your posture at your desk

Casting Couch Calf Raises
Try 3 sets of 10-15 reps, lift from chair or couch and return, then repeat this movement

V-Raise
Best in office move, this one move can work your upper body. Try with light weights to also help with posture. Do 2-3 sets of 10 reps

LIGHTS! CAMERA! ACTION! FITNESS!
NOW IS THE TIME TO GET BACK INTO THE FIT OF THINGS

Your biggest challenge right now is finding the time to fit it in. Plan your week according to your schedule and make adjustments.

AM- for the early bird
Midday- lunch hour
PM- for the late-nighter

Pick one of these time frames and get your cardio burn in

1. Treadmill/ 20 minutes/ increase incline
2. Stationary bike /20 minutes/ increase resistance
3. Elliptical trainer/ 20 minutes increase resistance or incline

Basic beginner workout
Start with 3 sets of 12 reps 2-3x a week
Remember to use a trainer to get you started

Lower Body
Lunges/ side lunges
Step-ups

Upper body
Bicep curl/free weight
Chest fly/ free weight
Triceps kickbacks
Front raise/ free weight
One arm row/ free weight

Abs/ 3 sets of 30 to start
Crunches/ reverse crunches

SAMPLE CIRCUIT PLAN
Dumbbell squats/ 20 reps
Dumbbell chess press/12 reps
Dumbbell row/ 12 reps
Calf raises/ 12 reps
Leg curls/ 12 reps
Triceps extension/ 12 reps
Bicep curls/ 12 reps
Crunches/ abs bench 25 reps
Start with 3 sets mix and match /adjust your weight or load accordingly

Now build your own hotlist of exercises to get you through the week
My hot list includes machines and cable exercises- my top contenders
Weighted dip machine- Assisted dips/ Assisted pullups
Cable hip adduction/ abduction
Cable pull/ external rotation
Cable pull through
Cable single arm triceps press down
Cable front raise
Cable bicep curl

10 FINAL CURTAIN CALL

THE FITNESS BREAKTHROUGH

Your next biggest challenge is to keep your fitness progressive. Performers continue to build your endurance to stay at peak performance. Now that you have mastered the three phases of the Modelsculptfitness Method- Model look, Model sculpt, Model bootcamp it's time to move to the final fitness curtain call.

PERFORMERS FITNESS BREAKTHROUGH
Keep your fitness workout challenging and stay at the top of your fitness game. Set fitness goals you can live with and expand your activities and sports. Include more adventurous outdoor activities
- Mountain climbing
- Hiking
- Triathlon
- Marathon
- Swimming
- Tennis
- Any new water sport or activity

Be creative and open yourself up to new fitness possibilities

USE THIS TIME TO WRITE YOUR OWN STORY SCRIPT!
Take time now to think about and describe your personal fit breakthrough.
Explore the changes you have made and what effect it has had on you and
your daily lifestyle.

YOUR FINAL STEP- THE MODELSCULPTFITNESS MAKEOVER
Last fitness quest, if you had to pick one new activity to try within the next
three months what would it be and why?
Identify three changes that you are going to make within the next 6
months?
List your best fitness traits
List what traits you want to change

Final test- remember to go review the 3 phases of the MSF method
1. Model look- getting the body ready. Focus on body alignment, abs
   & core conditioning and proper form
2. Model sculpt- try to focus on toning, tightening and defining your
   muscles through strength training
3. Model bootcamp- now focus on the high intensity workout include
   multi-joint exercises, plyometrics, sports drills, calisthenics

GET HOOKED 2 MODELSCULPTFITNESS!!!
In closing have fun with fitness!!!!
Make everyday a best workout day!
To all the actors, singers, dancers and performers stay upbeat and focused
with both your career aspirations and your lifetime fitness goals.

OPEN CALL
Although this workbook was primarily intended for actors and performers,
I encourage everyone to read and use this guide to becoming more fit. I
hope you will find the information helpful in your quest to developing a
more fit lifestyle.

To my readers feel free to use this workbook as a guide to create your
own favorite exercise routines, circuits, bootcamp workouts, personal
fitness tips and more. Look for my next workbook filled with fitness
worksheets and fitness breakdowns along with nutritional tips and casting
comfort foods. I have developed my second workbook as a follow up and
will contain handy fit sheets for you to use.

THAT'S A WRAP!!!
ENDING ON A HIGH NOTE!

Final thought
Again I stress that to make the best use of this workbook, always talk with your physician before doing any physical activity. Also, contact a fitness pro to conduct a fitness assessment and a series of fitness tests to determine your current fitness level.
This workbook is for motivational and educational information only. Do not attempt any exercises mentioned in this workbook before checking with your current physician, and working with a fitness professional. This workbook was designed to be used with a fitness trainer.

GET THE LOOK 2 GET BOOKED !
&
GET HOOKED 2 MODELSCULPTFITNESS!

MODELSCULPTFITNESS TERMS AND LINGO

Terms, lingo and meanings as described just for this workbook

M.O.D.E.L- my own daily exercise lifestyle

MSF-Modelsculptfitness

ACTOR-FITNESS-SWAG- an actor who knows they are at their peak performance of fitness

NET-WORKING-OUT- networking while working out

FITNESS BREAKDOWN- a breakdown of exercises to perform

MODEL BOOTCAMP - a fitness workout designed by you

CASTING COMFORT FOODS – tasty nutritional treats to enjoy before and after a workout

FITNESS BREAKTHROUGH -breaking through a fitness rut

WORKOUT DROP OUT - a performer who has ditched their workout routine

FITNESS LIGHTWEIGHT-someone who cannot handle a HIIT workout

STARVING ARTIST- a performer who does not eat enough foods with nutritional value

AUDITION YOUR NUTRITION-checking your nutrition and healthy choices on a regular basis

MOVES- exercises

PERFORMERS ENDURANCE/ PERFORMANCE PHILOSOPHY
A performer looking to increase stamina, energy and endurance to perform at a very high level of intensity for a long length of time

INDUSTRY LINGO! TAKE THE TIME AND DEFINE

IT'S TIME TO CHECK YOUR KNOWLEDGE ABOUT THE BIZ!

Actors and performers take the time and define the following terms as a refresher! Enjoy!

CALLBACK
GO SEE
AUDITION
AGENT
MANAGER
CASTING DIRECTOR
PRODUCER
CASTING CALL
OPEN CALL
SCRIPT
GREEN LIGHT
PILOT
HEADSHOT
ACTORS REEL
DEMO
ROUNDS
STATS
TEST SHOOT
VOUCHER
TRADE SHOW
COMMERCIAL COPY
COMMERCIAL PRINT
CATTLE CALL CASTING TYPE
BACK DROP
CUE CARDS
SCALE
SIDES
SPOT
CAMEO

LIST CONTINUED

TELEPROMPTER
ANIMATION
DUBBING
PSA
RESIDUAL
DAY RATE
FREELANCE
BOOKING OUT
CALL TIME
BILLING
COLD READING
HIATUS
PRINCIPAL ROLE
VOICEOVER
BACKGROUND
UNDERSTUDY
BLOCKING
SLATE
STAGED READING
SCREENPLAY
ACTING COACH
VOCAL COACH
SONGWRITER
CHOREOGRAPHER
PLAYWRIGHT
CINEMATOGRAPHER

ABOUT THE AUTHOR

Toni Renatta Hopper is a former Talent agent, Consultant, Producer and Author with over twenty years in the showbiz industry. As an Agent, she worked for a boutique agency in NY owned at the time by Elizabeth Taylor's daughter Maria Burton. Here she worked with many high profile and celebrity clients in television, film, and theatre. Her experience also includes ten years as the Director of the Barbizon Model agency and School in Highland Park overseeing the acting, modeling and talent center.

Her production experience includes many years as the Producer for the hit Actor Showcase Series. She is also the creator of the Modelsculptfitness brand that hosts networking and fitness events for actors and performers. As an avid fitness enthusiast she has written a fitness workbook series and is a Certified personal trainer and Certified sports nutritionist.

She received her B.A. from Wells College with a double bachelors in Russian Studies and History. She carries the distinction of being among a select few that holds a degree in that specialized field. She did graduate work at Hunter College in Russian Area Studies. She has also written a Monograph on the best Russian playwrights and novelists works for acting monologues.

www.ingramcontent.com/pod-product-compliance
Lightning Source LLC
Chambersburg PA
CBHW071120280526
45787CB00003B/1106